The Go-To KETO Chaffle Cooking Guide

Amazing Keto-friendly Chaffle Recipes To Lose Weight

Lily Sherman

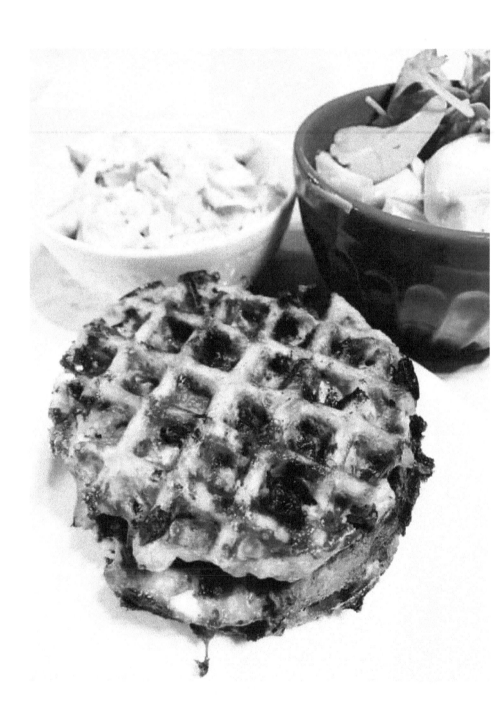

2

Table of contents

Asparagus Chaffle 7

Vegetarian Chaffle Sandwich 9

Ham and Cheese Chaffles Sandwich 11

Creamy Chicken Chaffle Sandwich 13

Mozzarella Panini 15

Turkey Patties & Vegetables Chaffles Sandwich 17

Cuban Sandwich Chaffle 19

Gourmet Chaffles Sandwich..21

U.S.A. Chaffles Sandwich 23

Big Chaffles Burger... 25

Tuna Chaffles Sandwich 28

Mexican Chaffles Sandwich 30

Avocado Chaffles Toast 32

Shrimps Green Chaffles Sandwich 34

Fish and Cajun Slaw Chaffles Sandwich... 36

Tex Chaffles Sandwich.. 39

Italian Chaffles Sandwich..41

Roast Beef Chaffles Sandwich 43

Turkey Chaffles Sandwich with Brie and Cranberry Jam 45

Egg and Bacon Chaffles Sandwich 47

Tasty Shrimps Chaffles Sandwich.. 49

Chaffles Sandwich with Sausage Patty 51

Worcestershire Beef Chaffles Sandwich 53

Delicious Bread Turkey Chaffles Sandwich 55

Trinidad Chaffles Sandwich 57

Veggie Chaffles Sandwich 59

Chaffles Sandwich with Turkey Patties 61

Mayonnaise and Ham Chaffles Sandwich 63

Blue Cheese Chaffles Sandwich 65

Ground Beef and Mushrooms Chaffles Sandwich 67

Butter, Spinach and Bacon Chaffles Sandwich 69

Avocado & Turkey Breast Chaffles Sandwich 71

Radishes Chaffles Toast 73

Ranch Chaffles Sandwich 75

Chicken & Radishes Chaffles Sandwich 77

Keto Ice Cream Sandwich Chaffle 79

Low Carb Mini Pizza Chaffle 81

Crabmeat Chaffles Sandwich 83

Grilled Chaffles Sandwich & Vegetables 85

Lemon Sauce Chicken Chaffles Sandwich 87

Sliced Beef Chaffles Sandwich 90

Fried Fish & Peppers Chaffles Sandwich 92

Cheese Peppers Chaffles Sandwich 94

Chaffles Sandwich Ham & Guacamole 96

Swiss Cheese and Salami Chaffles Sandwich 98

Strawberry Cream Sandwich Chaffles 100

5

Spicy Flavored Chaffle 102

Keto Chaffle With Cream 104

Sweet & Spicy Chaffle 106

Savory Herb Chaffle 108

Hot Brown Sandwich Chaffle 110

Asparagus Chaffle

Cooking: 15 Minutes

Servings: 4

Ingredients

Batter:

- 4 eggs
- 1½ cups grated mozzarella cheese
- ½ cup grated parmesan cheese
- 1 cup boiled asparagus, chopped
- Salt and pepper to taste
- ¼ cup almond flour
- 2 teaspns baking powder

Other:

- 2 tbsps cooking spray to brush your waffle maker
- ¼ cup Greek yogurt for serving
- ¼ cup chopped almonds for serving

Directions

1. Preheat now your waffle maker.

2. Add the eggs, grated mozzarella, grated parmesan, asparagus, salt and pepper, almond flour and baking powder to a bowl.
3. Mix with a fork.
4. Brush the heated waffle maker with cooking spray and add a few tbsps of the batter.
5. Close the lid and cook for about 7 minutes depending on your waffle maker.
6. Serve each chaffle with Greek yogurt and chopped almonds.

Nutrition:

Calories 316, Fat 24.9 g, Carbs 3 g, Sugar 1.2 g, Protein 18.2 g, Sodium 261 mg

Vegetarian Chaffle Sandwich

Cooking: 8 Minutes

Servings: 2

Ingredients

Chaffle:

- 1 large egg (beaten)
- 1/8 tsp onion powder
- 1 tbsp almond flour
- 1/2 cup shredded mozzarella cheese
- 1 tsp nutmeg
- 1/4 tsp baking powder

Sandwich Filling:

- 1/2 cup shredded carrot
- 1/2 cup sliced cucumber
- 1/2 medium bell pepper (sliced)
- 1 cup mixed salad greens
- 1/2 avocado (mashed and divided)
- 6 tbsp keto friendly hummus

Directions

For the chaffle:

1. Plug your waffle maker to Preheat now it. Spray it with non-stick cooking spray.
2. Combine the baking powder, nutmeg, flour and onion powder in a mixing bowl. Add the eggs and mix.
3. Add the cheese and mix well until the Ingredients are well combined and you have formed a smooth batter.
4. Pour the batter into your waffle maker and spread it out to the edges of your waffle maker to cover all the holes on it.
5. Close the waffle lid and cook for about 5 minutes or according to waffle maker's settings.
6. After the cooking cycle, remove now the chaffle from your waffle maker with a plastic or silicone utensil.
7. Add 3 tbsps of hummus to one chaffle and spread with a spoon for the sandwich.
8. Fill another chaffle with one half of the mashed avocado.
9. Fill the first chaffle slice with 1/4 cup sliced cucumber, 1/2 cup mixed salad greens, 1/4 cup shredded carrot and
10. one half of the sliced bell pepper.
11. Place the chaffle on top and press lightly.

12. Repeat step 7 to 10 for the remaining Ingredients to make the second sandwich.
13. Serve and enjoy.

Nutrition:

Fat 22g 28%, Carbohydrate 17.8g, 6% Sugars 4.6g, Protein 11.3g

Ham and Cheese Chaffles Sandwich

Preparation: 5 minutes

Cooking: 8 minutes

Servings: 2 chaffles

Ingredients

For chaffles:

- 1 egg
- ½ cup shredded mozzarella cheese
- Fresh basil to taste
- A pinch of salt and pepper

For filling:

- 1slice of ham

- 1 slice American cheese
- 1 tomato, sliced
- 1 lettuce leaf
- 1 tbsp keto butter

Directions

1. Heat up your waffle maker.
2. Add all the chaffles Ingredients to a tiny mixing bowl and combine well.
3. Pour half of the batter into your waffle maker and cook for 4 minutes until brown. Repeat now with the rest of the batter to make another chaffle.
4. Spread butter over the chaffle; top with a slice of ham, lettuce, tomato and American cheese. Cover with another chaffle.
5. Serve and enjoy!

Creamy Chicken Chaffle Sandwich

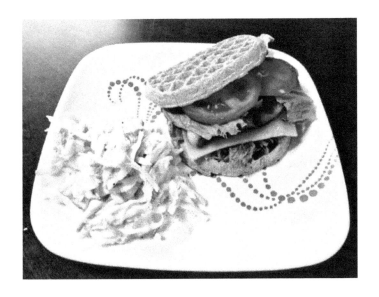

Cooking: 10 Minutes

Servings: 2

Ingredients

- Cooking spray
- 1 cup chicken breast fillet, cubed
- Salt and pepper to taste
- ¼ cup all-purpose cream
- 4 garlic chaffles
- Parsley, chopped

Directions

1. Spray your pan with oil.
2. Put it over medium heat.
3. Add the chicken fillet cubes.
4. Season with salt and pepper.
5. Reduce heat and add the cream.
6. Spread chicken mixture on top of the chaffle.
7. Garnish with parsley and top with another chaffle.

Nutrition:

Calories 273, Total Fat 34g, Saturated Fat 4.1g, Cholesterol 62mg, Sodium 373 mg, Total Carbohydrate 22.5g, Dietary Fiber 1.1g, Total Sugars 3.2g, Protein 17.5g, Potassium 177 mg

Mozzarella Panini

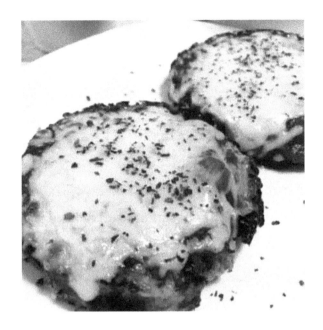

Preparation: 15 minutes

Cooking: 15 minutes

Servings: 1

Ingredients

- Classic Chaffle Recipe

Sandwich Filling

- 1 ounce of of mozzarella, thinly sliced

- 1 heirloom tomato, thinly sliced
- 1/4 of a cup of pesto
- 2 fresh basil leaves

Directions

1. Follow the Classic Chaffle recipe.
2. Once the chaffles are done, lay two side by side.
3. Spread the pesto on one, then layer the Mozzarella cheese and tomatoes and sandwich together.

Nutrition:

Net Carbs: 2g, Calories: 234, Total Fat: 14.7g, Saturated Fat: 2g, Protein: 23.3g, Carbs: 2.1g, Fiber: 0.1g, Sugar: 2g

Turkey Patties & Vegetables Chaffles Sandwich

Preparation: 10 minutes

Cooking: 30 minutes

Servings: 4 chaffles

Ingredients

For Chaffles:

- 2 eggs, beaten
- 1 cup cheddar cheese, shredded
- A pinch of salt and pepper

For Patties and Filling:

- 2 cups ground turkey
- Lettuce leaves
- 1 tomato, sliced
- 1 onion, sliced and browned
- 1 sliced grilled zucchini
- Keto BBQ sauce
- 1 tbsp olive oil
- A pinch of salt and pepper

Directions

For the Chaffles:

1. Heat up your waffle maker.
2. Add all the chaffles Ingredients to a tiny mixing bowl and stir until well combined.
3. Pour ¼ of the batter into your waffle maker and cook for 4 minutes until golden brown. Repeat now with the rest of the batter to prepare the other chaffles.
4. Let cool for 3 minutes to let chaffles get crispy.

For the Patties:

5. In a tiny bowl, season the ground turkey with salt and pepper.
6. Create tiny patties.
7. In a saucepan over low heat, cook the turkey patties in olive oil until completely cooked and brown.

For Topping:

8. Spread each chaffle with Keto BBQ sauce. Garnish with lettuce, tomato, onion, zucchini and the patty. Cover with another chaffle.
9. Serve and enjoy!

Cuban Sandwich Chaffle

Preparation: 15 minutes

Cooking: 15 minutes

Servings: 1

Ingredients

- Classic Chaffle Recipe

Cubano:

- 1/4 of a pound of ham, cooked and sliced
- 1/4 of a pound of pork, roasted and sliced
- 1/4-pound Swiss cheese, thinly sliced
- 3 dill pickles, sliced in half

Directions

1. Follow the Classic Chaffle recipe.
2. Take two chaffles and lay side by side.
3. Lay on the meat, cheese, and pickles.
4. Sandwich the two chaffles together.
5. Put the sandwich in a to aster oven if you want it hot.
6. Heat for 5 minutes or until cheese is Melt nowed.

Nutrition:

Net Carbs: 4.8g, Calories: 323, Total Fat: 51.5g, Saturated Fat: 23.3g, Protein: 41.3g, Carbs: 7g, Fiber: 2.2g, Sugar: 2.3g

Gourmet Chaffles Sandwich

Preparation: 5 minutes

Cooking: 8 minutes

Servings: 2 chaffles

Ingredients

For the Chaffles:

- 1 egg
- ½ cup shredded Cheddar cheese

For the Sandwich:

- 2 strips bacon
- 1-2 slices tomato
- 1-2 lettuce leaves
- 1 tbsp mayonnaise

Directions

1. Heat up your waffle maker.
2. Mix egg and shredded cheese in a tiny mixing bowl.

3. Pour half of the batter into your waffle maker and cook for 4 minutes. Repeat now with the rest of the batter to make another chaffle.
4. Let cool for 3 minutes to let chaffles get crispy.
5. In a pan over medium heat, cook the bacon until crispy.
6. Assemble the sandwich topping the chaffle with bacon, lettuce, tomato, and mayonnaise.
7. Serve and enjoy!

U.S.A. Chaffles Sandwich

Preparation: 5 minutes

Cooking: 8 minutes

Servings: 2 chaffles

Ingredients

For the Chaffles:

- 1 egg
- ½ cup shredded Cheddar cheese

For the Sandwich:

- 2 strips bacon
- 1 egg
- 1-2 slices tomato
- 1 slice American cheese

Directions

1. Heat up your waffle maker.
2. Mix egg and shredded cheese in a tiny mixing bowl.
3. Pour half of the batter into your waffle maker and cook for 4 minutes. Repeat now with the rest of the batter to make another chaffle.

4. Let cool for 3 minutes to let chaffles get crispy.

5. In a pan over medium heat, cook the bacon until crispy.

6. In the same skillet, in 1 tbsp of reserved bacon drippings, fry the egg over medium heat.

7. Assemble the sandwich, serve and enjoy!

Big Chaffles Burger

Preparation: 9 minutes

Cooking: 20 minutes

Servings: 4 chaffles

Ingredients

For the Chaffles:

- 2 eggs
- 1 cup shredded mozzarella cheese
- ¼ tsp garlic powder

For the Cheeseburgers:

- ½ cup ground beef
- ½ tsp garlic powder
- 2 slices American cheese

For the Sauce:

- 2 tsp mayonnaise
- 1 tsp ketchup
- 1 tsp dill pickle relish

To Assemble:

- 1-2 lettuce leaves, shredded

- 2 dill pickles
- 1 tsp onion, minced

Directions

To make the Burgers:

1. Heat a skillet over medium heat.
2. Divide the ground beef into 2 balls and place each on the grill. Let cook for 1 minute.
3. Flatten the meat and sprinkle it with garlic powder.
4. Cook 2 minutes or until halfway cooked through. Flip the burgers carefully and sprinkle with remaining garlic powder. Continue cooking until cooked through.
5. Place one slice of cheese over each burger and then stack the burgers and set aside.

To make the chaffles and Assemble the burger:

6. Heat up your waffle maker.
7. Mix now the egg, cheese, and garlic powder in a tiny mixing bowl.
8. Pour ¼ of the batter into your waffle maker and cook for 4 minutes. Repeat now with the rest of the batter to make the other chaffles.
9. Prepare the sauce whisking together all the Ingredients.

10. Top one chaffle with the stacked burger patties, shredded lettuce, pickles, and onions. Cover with another chaffle.
11. Serve with the sauce and enjoy!

Tuna Chaffles Sandwich

Preparation: 10 minutes

Cooking: 8 minutes

Servings: 2 chaffles

Ingredients

For Chaffles:

- 1 egg, beaten
- 1 cup tomatoes, chopped
- ¼ cup parmesan cheese, shredded
- ½ cup swiss cheese, shredded
- 1 tsp fresh basil
- A pinch of salt and pepper

For Filling:

- A can of drained tuna
- Lettuce leaf
- 1 tbsp keto mayonnaise

Directions

1. Heat up your waffle maker.

28

2. Add all the chaffles Ingredients except for parmesan cheese to a tiny mixing bowl and combine well.

3. Pour half of the batter into your waffle maker, sprinkle with 1-2 tbsp of shredded parmesan cheese and cook for 4 minutes. Repeat now with the rest of the batter to make another chaffle.

4. Let cool for 3 minutes to let chaffles get crispy.

5. Spread the chaffle with keto mayonnaise, top with drained tuna, a lettuce leaf and cover with the other chaffle.

6. Serve and enjoy!

Mexican Chaffles Sandwich

Preparation: 15 minutes

Cooking: 8 minutes

Servings: 2 chaffles

Ingredients

For the Chaffles:

- 1 cup mozzarella cheese, grated
- 2 eggs
- A pinch of salt
- Spices to taste
- 2 slices chorizo for the filling, very thin

For the Avocado Cream:

- 1 tiny avocado pulp, mashed
- 1 tbsp cherry tomatoes, diced
- 1 tsp onions, sliced
- 2 tbsp olive oil
- 1 tbsp lemon juice
- A pinch of salt and pepper
- A pinch of Chili powder

Directions

For the Avocado Cream:

1. In a tiny bowl, add the olive oil and lemon juice to the avocado and stir.
2. Add onions, and tomatoes, mix well and season with salt, pepper, and chili to taste.

For the Chaffles:

3. Heat up your waffle maker.
4. Add all the chaffles Ingredients except chorizo to a tiny mixing bowl. Stir until well combined.
5. Pour half of the batter into your waffle maker and cook for 4 minutes. Repeat now with the rest of the batter to make another chaffle.
6. Let cool for 3 minutes to let chaffles get crispy.
7. Spread avocado cream on a chaffle and cover with chorizo, then put another chaffle on top.
8. Serve and enjoy!

Avocado Chaffles Toast

Preparation: 5 minutes

Cooking: 16 minutes

Servings: 4 chaffles

Ingredients

For Chaffles:

- 2 eggs
- 1 cup cheese, shredded
- 4 tbsp avocado, pulp
- 1 tsp lemon juice
- A pinch of salt and pepper

For Topping:

- 2 eggs
- ½ avocado, sliced
- 1 tomato, sliced

Directions

1. Combine the avocado pulp with lemon juice, salt and pepper in a tiny mixing bowl.

2. Beat the eggs with the avocado cream.

3. Heat up your waffle maker.

4. Pour ¼ of the batter into your waffle maker and cook for 4 minutes until golden brown. Repeat now with the rest of the batter to make the other chaffles.

5. Let cool for 3 minutes to let chaffles get crispy.

6. In the meantime, in a tiny saucepan fry the eggs.

7. Top every chaffle with fried egg, tomatoes and avocado slices. Cover with another chaffle.

8. Serve and enjoy!

Shrimps Green Chaffles Sandwich

Preparation: 15 minutes

Cooking: 24 minutes

Servings: 8 chaffles

Ingredients

For Chaffles:

- 4 eggs, beaten
- 2 cups mozzarella cheese, shredded
- 1 tsp your favorite spices

Ingredients for filling:

- 4 tbsp shrimps, deveined and cooked
- 4 slices bacon cooked
- 1 avocado, sliced
- ¼ cup onion, sliced
- A pinch of salt and pepper

Directions

<u>For Chaffles:</u>

1. Heat up the mini waffle maker.
2. Add all the chaffles Ingredients to a tiny mixing bowl and stir until well combined.
3. Pour 1/8 of the batter into your waffle maker and cook for 4 minutes. Repeat now with the rest of the batter to make the other chaffles.
4. Let cool for 3 minutes to let chaffles get crispy.

<u>Assemble the Sandwich:</u>

5. Top the chaffle with a slice of bacon, shrimps, avocado and onion. Add salt, pepper and your favorite spices to taste. Cover with another chaffle.
6. Serve with keto mayonnaise or sour cream and enjoy!

Fish and Cajun Slaw Chaffles Sandwich

Preparation: 12 minutes

Cooking: 26 minutes

Servings: 4 chaffles

Ingredients

For Chaffles:

- 2 eggs, beaten
- 2 tbsp almond flour
- 2 tbsp full-fat plain Greek yogurt
- ¼ tsp baking powder
- 1 cup shredded cheddar cheese

For Cajun Slaw:

- 1 cup coleslaw
- 3 tbsp keto mayonnaise
- 1 tbsp Greek yogurt
- 1 tsp Tabasco sauce
- ½ tsp Cajun seasoning

For Fish:

- ¼ cup avocado oil

- 2 tiny flounder
- ¼ cup heavy cream
- ½ tsp lemon juice
- 1/3 cup of shredded parmesan cheese
- 1/3 cup of pork rind crumbs
- ½ tsp garlic powder
- A pinch of black pepper

Directions

For Chaffles:

1. Heat up the mini waffle maker.
2. Mix all the chaffles Ingredients to a tiny mixing bowl and stir until well combined.
3. Pour ¼ of the batter into your waffle maker and cook for 4 minutes. Repeat now with the rest of the batter to make the other chaffles.
4. Let cool for 3 minutes to let chaffles get crispy.

For Cajun Slaw:

5. Add all the Ingredients to a tiny bowl and mix well.

For Fish:

6. In a saucepan heat oil over medium-high heat.
7. Mix now the heavy cream and lemon juice in a tiny bowl until it thickens.

8. In a separate bowl, combine the parmesan cheese, pork rind crumbs, garlic powder, and pepper until mixed.

9. Dip the fish filet in the cream mixture, then sprinkle with crumbs.

10. Place it into the oil and Repeat now with the remaining fish filet. Cook for about 5 min, until golden brown.

Assemble the Chaffles Sandwich:

11. Top the chaffle with a fish filet, the slaw, and then top with another chaffle.

12. Serve and enjoy!

Tex Chaffles Sandwich

Preparation: 5 minutes

Cooking: 40 minutes

Servings: 10 chaffles

Ingredients

For the Chaffles:

- 4 eggs, beaten
- ¼ cup almond flour
- 4 tbsp cream cheese
- ½ tsp baking powder
- 2 tsp yellow flax seed meal
- 2 cups mozzarella cheese, shredded

For the Sandwich:

- 5 hard-boiled eggs, sliced
- 5 slices bacon
- 5 slices American cheese

Directions

1. Heat up the mini waffle maker.

2. Combine the raw eggs with the almond flour, cream cheese, baking powder and blend until smoothy.

3. Sprinkle 1/10 teaspn of the flax seed meal and 1 tbspn of mozzarella onto your waffle maker. Add two tbsps of egg mixture and cook for 4 minutes. Repeat now with the rest of the batter to prepare the other chaffles.

4. Let cool for 3 minutes to let chaffles get crispy.

5. Top the chaffle with bacon, a few slices of hard-boiled egg, American cheese and cover with another chaffle.

6. Serve and enjoy!

Italian Chaffles Sandwich

Preparation: 5 minutes

Cooking: 16 minutes

Servings: 4 chaffles

Ingredients

For the Chaffles:

- 2 large eggs, beaten
- 1 cup shredded cheddar cheese

For the Filling:

- 1 tomato, sliced
- 2 lettuce leaves
- 1 cup mozzarella cheese, shredded
- 2 tbsp keto mayonnaise
- 1 tsp of dried oregano

Directions

For the Chaffles:

1. Heat up your waffle maker.

2. Add egg and shredded cheese to a tiny mixing bowl and combine well.
3. Pour ¼ of the batter into your waffle maker and cook for 4 minutes. Repeat now with the rest of the batter to prepare the remaining chaffles.
4. Let cool for 3 minutes to let chaffles get crispy.
5. Spread the chaffle with keto mayo. Top with a slice of tomato, a lettuce leaf, and sprinkle with dried oregano and mozzarella cheese. Cover with another chaffle.
6. Serve and enjoy!

Roast Beef Chaffles Sandwich

Preparation: 5 minutes

Cooking: 16 minutes

Servings: 4 chaffles

Ingredients

For the Chaffles:

- 2 large eggs
- 1 cup shredded cheddar cheese
- A pinch of salt

For the Filling:

- 1 tomato, sliced
- 2 lettuce leaves
- 2 thin slices of Roast beef
- 2 tbsp keto mayonnaise

Directions

For the Chaffles:

1. Heat up your waffle maker.

2. Add eggs, shredded cheese and salt to a tiny mixing bowl and combine well.

3. Pour ¼ of the batter into your waffle maker and cook for 4 minutes. Repeat now with the rest of the batter to prepare the remaining chaffles.

4. Let cool for 3 minutes to let chaffles get crispy.

5. Spread the chaffle with keto mayo. Top with a slice of tomato, lettuce leave and roast beef. Cover with another chaffle.

6. Serve and enjoy!

Turkey Chaffles Sandwich with Brie and Cranberry Jam

Preparation: 4 minutes

Cooking: 8 minutes

Servings: 2 chaffles

Ingredients

For the Chaffles:

- 1 large egg, beaten
- ½ cup mozzarella cheese, shredded
- 2 tbsp almond flour

For the Filling:

- 1slice of turkey
- 1 slice of Brie cheese
- 1 tbsp chia cranberry jam

Directions

For the Chaffles:

1. Heat up your waffle maker.

2. Add all the chaffles Ingredients to a tiny mixing bowl and combine well.

3. Pour half of the batter into your waffle maker and cook for 4 minutes until golden brown. Repeat now with the rest of the batter to prepare the remaining chaffle.

4. Let cool for 3 minutes to let chaffles get crispy.

5. Spread the chaffle with chia cranberry jam and top with a slice of brie and of turkey.

6. Add spices if desired. Cover with another chaffle.

7. Serve and enjoy!

Egg and Bacon Chaffles Sandwich

Preparation: 4 minutes

Cooking: 16 minutes

Servings: 4 chaffles

Ingredients

For the Chaffles:

- 2 large eggs
- 1 cup shredded cheddar cheese
- A pinch of salt

For the Filling:

- 2 hard-boiled eggs, sliced
- 2 lettuce leaves
- 4 slices of bacon, fried
- 2 tbsp keto mayonnaise or keto ketchup

Directions

For the Chaffles:

1. Heat up your waffle maker.

2. Add eggs, shredded cheese and salt to a tiny mixing bowl and combine well.

3. Pour ¼ of the batter into your waffle maker and cook for 4 minutes until brown. Repeat now with the rest of the batter to prepare the remaining chaffles.

4. Let cool for 3 minutes to let chaffles get crispy.

5. Spread the chaffle with keto mayo or keto ketchup. Top with lettuce leave, bacon, hard-boiled egg and add spices if desired. Cover with another chaffle.

6. Serve and enjoy!

Tasty Shrimps Chaffles Sandwich

Preparation: 5 minutes

Cooking: 16 minutes

Servings: 4 chaffles

Ingredients

For shrimps:

- 1 tsp olive oil
- 2 tbsp shrimps, peeled and deveined
- 1 tbsp Creole seasoning
- 2 tbsp hot sauce
- 3 tbsp butter
- A pinch of salt

For the Chaffles:

- 2 eggs, beaten
- 1 cup Monterey Jack cheese, shredded

For Filling:

- 1 tomato, sliced
- 2 tbsp keto mayonnaise

Directions

For shrimps:

1. In a tiny saucepan over medium heat, heat the olive oil and cook the shrimps for approx. 3-4 minutes.
2. Season the shrimps with Creole seasoning.
3. Pour in the butter and the hot sauce. Mix well.

For the Chaffles:

4. Heat up your waffle maker.
5. Add all the chaffles Ingredients to a tiny mixing bowl and stir until well combined.
6. Pour ¼ of the batter into your waffle maker and cook for 4 minutes until golden brown. Repeat now with the rest of the batter to make the other chaffles.
7. Let cool for 3 minutes to let chaffles get crispy.
8. Spread the chaffle with keto mayonnaise, a slice of tomato and the shrimps. Cover with another chaffle.
9. Serve and enjoy!

Chaffles Sandwich with Sausage Patty

Preparation: 10 minutes

Cooking: 16 minutes

Servings: 4 chaffles

Ingredients

For the Chaffles:

- 2 large eggs, beaten
- 1 cup mozzarella cheese, shredded
- 2 tbsp coconut flour
- 2 tbsp keto mayonnaise
- ½ tsp baking powder

For the filling:

- 2 sausage patties, cooked
- 2 slices of cheddar cheese
- A pinch of salt and pepper

Directions

For Chaffles:

1. Heat up your waffle maker.

2. Add all the Ingredients for the chaffles to a tiny mixing bowl and combine well.
3. Pour ¼ of the batter into your waffle maker and cook for 4 minutes until golden brown. Repeat now with the rest of the batter to prepare other chaffles.
4. Top each chaffle with a slice of cheddar cheese, a sausage patty and a pinch of salt and pepper. Cover with the other chaffle.
5. Serve and enjoy!

Worcestershire Beef Chaffles Sandwich

Preparation: 10 minutes

Cooking: 8 minutes

Servings: 2 chaffles

Ingredients

For beef:

- ½ cup beef broth
- 4 oz roast beef, very thin

For Chaffles:

- 1 large egg, beaten
- 1 tsp coconut flour
- ¼ tsp baking powder
- ½ cup cheese, shredded

For sauce:

- 1 tbsp keto ketchup
- ¼ tsp Worcestershire sauce
- A pinch of pepper

Directions

For beef:

1. In a big pan bring to a boil the beef broth.
2. Cook the beef on the broth over low heat for approx. 5 minutes.
3. Set aside.

For sauce:

4. Combine all the sauce Ingredients in a tiny mixing bowl.

For Chaffles:

5. Heat up your waffle maker.
6. Add all the chaffles Ingredients to a tiny mixing bowl and stir until well combined.
7. Pour half of the batter into your waffle maker and cook for 4 minutes until brown. Repeat now with the rest of the batter to make another chaffle.
8. Spread the chaffle with the sauce and top with the beef. Cover with another chaffle.
9. Serve and enjoy!

Delicious Bread Turkey Chaffles Sandwich

Preparation: 5 minutes

Cooking: 8 minutes

Servings: 2 chaffles

Ingredients

For Chaffles:

- 2 eggs white, beaten
- 2 tbsp almond flour
- 1 tbsp mayonnaise
- ¼ tsp baking powder
- 1 tsp water
- Salt to taste

Ingredients for the filling:

- 1 tbsp keto mayonnaise
- 1 slice deli ham
- 1 slice deli turkey
- 1 slice cheddar cheese
- 1 lettuce leaf

- 1 tomato, sliced

Directions

1. Heat up your waffle maker.
2. Add all the Ingredients to a tiny mixing bowl and stir until well combined.
3. Pour half of the batter into your waffle maker and cook for 4 minutes until golden brown. Repeat now with the rest of the batter to make another chaffle.
4. Spread each chaffle with mayonnaise, top with tomato slice, the lettuce leaf, a slice of cheddar cheese, ham and turkey. Cover with another chaffle.
5. Serve immediately and enjoy!

Trinidad Chaffles Sandwich

Preparation: 5 minutes

Cooking: 8 minutes

Servings: 2 chaffles

Ingredients

For Chaffles:

- 1 egg, beaten
- 1 tbsp almond flour
- 1 tbsp Greek yogurt
- 1/8 tsp baking powder
- ¼ cup swiss cheese, shredded

For filling:

- 3 ounce ofs roast pork
- 1 slice deli ham
- 1 slice swiss cheese
- 4 pickles, minced
- 1 tsp keto mustard

Directions

1. Heat up your waffle maker.

2. Add all the chaffles Ingredients to a tiny mixing bowl and stir until well combined.
3. Pour half of the batter into your waffle maker and cook for 4 minutes until golden brown. Repeat now with the rest of the batter to make another chaffle.
4. Let cool for 3 minutes to let chaffles get crispy.
5. Spread the chaffle with mustard and top with Ingredients in this order: roast pork, swiss cheese, deli ham, pickles. Cover with another chaffle.
6. Microwave the chaffles for 20 seconds and serve immediately. Enjoy!

Veggie Chaffles Sandwich

Preparation: 5 minutes

Cooking: 8 minutes

Servings: 2 chaffles

Ingredients

For Chaffles:

- 1 egg
- ½ cup mozzarella cheese, shredded
- ½ cup zucchini, grated
- ½ tbsp onion, minced
- ½ tbsp tomato, diced
- 1 garlic clove, minced
- Fresh dill, chopped
- A pinch of salt

For filling:

- Lettuce leaves
- 1 tbsp keto mayonnaise
- 1 slice cheddar cheese

Directions

1. Heat up your waffle maker.

2. Whisk eggs in bowl and stir in zucchini, onions, garlic, herbs, tomatoes and most of the cheese. You can reserve some of the cheese to make the crispy coating.

3. Pour half of the batter into your waffle maker and cook for 4 minutes until brown. Repeat now with the rest of the batter to make another chaffle.

4. Let cool for 3 minutes to let chaffles get crispy.

5. Spread the chaffle with keto mayonnaise and top with lettuce and cheddar cheese. Cover with another chaffle.

6. Serve and enjoy!

Chaffles Sandwich with Turkey Patties

Preparation: 10 minutes

Cooking: 30 minutes

Servings: 4 chaffles

Ingredients

For Chaffles:

- 2 eggs, beaten
- 1 cup cheddar cheese, shredded
- A pinch of salt and pepper

For Patties and Filling:

- 2 cups ground turkey
- Lettuce leaves
- 1 tomato, sliced
- Keto Ketchup & Keto Mayonnaise
- 1 tbsp olive oil
- A pinch of salt and pepper

Directions

<u>For the Chaffles:</u>

1. Heat up your waffle maker.
2. Add all the chaffles Ingredients to a tiny mixing bowl and stir until well combined.
3. Pour ¼ of the batter into your waffle maker and cook for 4 minutes until golden brown. Repeat now with the rest of the batter to prepare the other chaffles.
4. Let cool for 3 minutes to let chaffles get crispy.

<u>For the Patties:</u>

5. In a tiny bowl, season the ground turkey with salt and pepper.
6. Create tiny patties.
7. In a saucepan over low heat, cook the turkey patties in olive oil until completely cooked and brown.

<u>For Topping:</u>

8. Top each chaffle with Keto mayo or Keto Ketchup according to your taste. Garnish with lettuce, tomato and the patty. Cover with another chaffle.
9. Serve and enjoy!

Mayonnaise and Ham Chaffles Sandwich

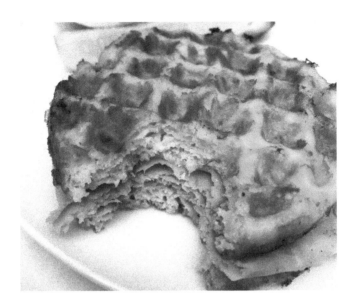

Preparation: 5 minutes

Cooking: 16 minutes

Servings: 4 chaffles

Ingredients

For Chaffles:

- 2 large eggs, beaten
- 2 tbsp keto mayonnaise
- ½ tbsp almond flour

- 1 tbsp cream cheese
- A pinch of salt and pepper

<u>For filling:</u>

- Lettuce leaves
- 1 tomato sliced
- 2 slices of ham
- 1 scallion, sliced and browned
- Keto Ketchup

Directions

1. Heat up your waffle maker.
2. Add all the Ingredients to a tiny mixing bowl and stir until well combined.
3. Pour ¼ of the batter into your waffle maker and cook for 4 minutes until brown. Repeat now with the rest of the batter to make the other chaffles.
4. Let cool for 3 minutes to let chaffles get crispy.
5. Spread the chaffle with keto ketchup. Garnish with lettuce, tomato, ham and onions. Cover with another chaffle.
6. Serve warm and enjoy!

Blue Cheese Chaffles Sandwich

Preparation: 5 minutes

Cooking: 8 minutes

Servings: 2 chaffles

Ingredients

For Chaffles:

- 1 large egg, beaten
- ½ cup mozzarella cheese, shredded
- ¼ cup blue cheese, shredded
- 1 tsp sweetener

For filling:

- 1 tbsp raspberries jam
- Lettuce leaves
- 1-2 slices of deli ham

Directions

For Chaffles:

1. Heat up your waffle maker.

2. Add all the Ingredients to a tiny mixing bowl and stir until well combined.
3. Pour half of the batter into your waffle maker and cook for 4 minutes until golden brown. Repeat now with the rest of the batter to make another chaffle.
4. Let cool for 3 minutes to let chaffles get crispy.
5. Spread the chaffle with raspberries jam. Garnish with a lettuce leaf and a slice of deli ham.
6. Cover with another chaffle.
7. Serve and enjoy!

Ground Beef and Mushrooms Chaffles Sandwich

Preparation: 5 minutes

Cooking: 20 minutes

Servings: 2 chaffles

Ingredients

For Chaffles:

- 1 egg, beaten
- ½ cup shredded cheddar cheese
- ½ tbsp fresh basil, finely chopped
- A pinch of salt

For beef:

- 1 tsp olive oil
- 2 cups ground beef
- ½ tsp garlic powder
- 1 onion, chopped
- 2 tbsp white mushrooms, chopped
- 1 tsp butter for topping

Directions

<u>For Chaffles:</u>

1. Heat up your waffle maker.
2. Add egg, shredded cheddar cheese, a pinch of salt and basil to a tiny mixing bowl and combine well.
3. Pour half of the batter into your waffle maker and cook for 4 minutes until brown. Repeat now with the rest of the batter to make another chaffle.

<u>For beef:</u>

4. In a saucepan over medium heat cook the ground beef in olive oil. Season with salt and pepper if needed and add mushrooms and onion. Stir occasionally and cook until the meat is browned.

<u>For Topping:</u>

5. Spread the chaffle with butter and garnish with beef and mushrooms. Cover with another chaffle.
6. Serve immediately and enjoy!

Butter, Spinach and Bacon Chaffles Sandwich

Preparation: 5 minutes

Cooking: 8 minutes

Servings: 2 chaffles

Ingredients

For Chaffles:

- 1 large egg, beaten
- ½ cup of mozzarella cheese, shredded
- 2 tbsp almond flour
- ¼ tsp baking powder
- A pinch of salt

For Topping:

- 2 fresh spinach leaves
- 1 tbsp butter
- 1 tsp parmesan cheese, flakes
- 1 slices of bacon, cooked

Directions

1. Heat up your waffle maker.

2. Add all the Ingredients to a tiny mixing bowl and combine well.

3. Pour half of the batter into your waffle maker and cook for 4 minutes until brown. Repeat now with the rest of the batter to make another chaffle.

4. Let cool for 3 minutes to let chaffles get crispy.

5. Spread the chaffle with butter. Garnish with spinach leaves and bacon. Sprinkle with parmesan flakes. Cover with another chaffle.

6. Serve and enjoy!

Avocado & Turkey Breast Chaffles Sandwich

Preparation: 15 minutes

Cooking: 8 minutes

Servings: 2 chaffles

Ingredients

For the Chaffles:

- 1 cup mozzarella cheese, grated
- 2 eggs, beaten
- A pinch of salt
- Spices to taste
- 1 slice turkey breast for the filling, very thin
- 1 tsp keto mayonnaise for the filling

For the avocado cream:

- 1 tiny avocado pulp, mashed
- 1 tbsp cherry tomatoes, diced
- 1 tsp onions, sliced
- 2 tbsp olive oil
- 1 tbsp lemon juice

- A pinch of salt and pepper
- A pinch of Chili powder

Directions

For the avocado cream:

1. In a tiny bowl, add the olive oil and lemon juice to the avocado and stir.
2. Add onions, and tomatoes, mix well and season with salt, pepper, and chili to taste.

For the Chaffles:

3. Heat up your waffle maker.
4. Add all the chaffles Ingredients except turkey breast and mayonnaise to a tiny mixing bowl. Stir until well combined.
5. Pour half of the batter into your waffle maker and cook for 4 minutes. Repeat now with the rest of the batter to make another chaffle.
6. Let cool for 3 minutes to let chaffles get crispy.
7. Spread avocado cream on a chaffle, fill with turkey breast. Spread keto mayonnaise on the other chaffle and close the sandwich.
8. Serve and enjoy!

Radishes Chaffles Toast

Preparation: 5 minutes

Cooking: 8 minutes

Servings: 2 chaffles

Ingredients

For Chaffles:

- 1 large egg, beaten
- ½ cup mozzarella cheese, shredded
- ½ tsp baking powder
- 2 tbsp radishes, boiled and puree
- A pinch of black pepper

For Topping:

- 1 tbsp butter
- 1 slice of bacon, browned
- 2 fresh spinach leaves
- 1 tsp parmesan cheese, shredded

Directions:

1. Heat up your waffle maker.

2. Add all the chaffles Ingredients to a tiny mixing bowl and stir until well combined.
3. Pour half of the batter into your waffle maker and cook for 4 minutes until golden brown. Repeat now with the rest of the batter to make another chaffle.
4. Let cool for 3 minutes to let chaffles get crispy.
5. Spread the chaffle with butter, top with bacon, spinach leaves and sprinkle with parmesan cheese. Cover with another chaffle.
6. Serve and enjoy!

Ranch Chaffles Sandwich

Preparation: 5 minutes

Cooking: 8 minutes

Servings: 2 chaffles

Ingredients

For Chaffles:

- 1 egg, beaten
- ½ cup cheddar cheese, shredded
- ¼ cup chicken cooked, shredded
- 1 tbsp bacon bits, browned
- 1 tsp Ranch seasoning

For filling:

- Lettuce leaves
- 1 tiny tomato, sliced
- 1 tsp dried oregano
- 1 slice of American cheese

Directions

1. Heat up your waffle maker.

2. Add all the chaffles Ingredients to a tiny mixing bowl and stir until well combined.
3. Pour half of the batter into your waffle maker and cook for 4 minutes until golden brown. Repeat now with the rest of the batter to make another chaffle.
4. Top the chaffle with lettuce, tomato slices, oregano and a slice of American cheese. Cover with another chaffle.
5. Serve warm and enjoy!

Chicken & Radishes Chaffles Sandwich

Preparation: 5 minutes

Cooking: 8 minutes

Servings: 2 chaffles

Ingredients

For Chaffles:

- 1 egg, beaten
- ½ cup cheddar cheese, shredded

For filling:

- Lettuce leaves
- ¼ cup chicken cooked, shredded
- 1 tbsp radishes, grilled and thin sliced
- 1 tbsp cream cheese, softened

Directions

1. Heat up your waffle maker.
2. Add all the chaffles Ingredients to a tiny mixing bowl and stir until well combined.

3. Pour half of the batter into your waffle maker and cook for 4 minutes until golden brown. Repeat now with the rest of the batter to make another chaffle.

4. Spread the chaffle with cream cheese. Top with lettuce, chicken and grilled radishes. Cover with another chaffle.

5. Serve warm and enjoy!

Keto Ice Cream Sandwich Chaffle

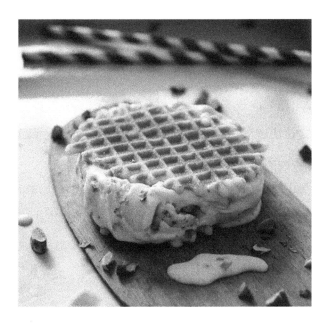

Preparation: 5 minutes

Cooking: 5 minutes

Servings: 2

Ingredients

- 2 Tbs cocoa
- 2 Tbs Monkfruit Confectioner's
- 1 egg
- 1/4 teaspn baking powder

- 1 Tbs Heavy Whipped Cream
- Add selected keto ice cream

Directions

1. Whip the egg in a tiny bowl.
2. Add the rest of the Ingredients and mix well until smooth and creamy.
3. Pour half of the batter into a mini waffle maker and cook until fully cooked for 2 1/2 to 3 minutes.
4. Allow the ice cream to cool completely before ice cream is placed in the center.
5. Freeze to solid.
6. Serve and bear the weather!

Low Carb Mini Pizza Chaffle

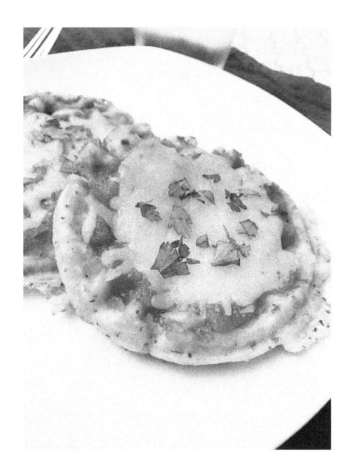

Preparation: 5 minutes

Cooking: 5 minutes

Servings: 2

Ingredients

- 1 egg
- 1/2 cup mozzarella cheese shredded
- 1/4 teaspn of garlic powder
- 1/2 tsp Italian seasoning
- Salt and pepper

Toppings:

- Tomato sauce, cheese, pepperoni, etc

Directions:

1. Put all Ingredients in a bowl. Mix well.
2. Preheat now your waffle maker. When it's hot, spray olive oil, put half of the dough in a mini waffle maker, or put all dough in a large waffle maker. Cook each chaffle for 2-4 minutes.
3. Add the toppings and bake or fry the mini pizza until the cheese topping has Melt nowed. Serve and enjoy!

Crabmeat Chaffles Sandwich

Preparation: 5 minutes

Cooking: 8 minutes

Servings: 2 chaffles

Ingredients

For Chaffles:

- 1 large egg, beaten
- ½ cup of mozzarella cheese, shredded
- 2 tbsp almond flour
- ¼ tsp baking powder
- ¼ tsp garlic powder

For filling:

- ¾ cup crabmeat
- 1 tbsp keto mayonnaise
- 1 tsp lemon juice
- Lettuce leaves
- 1 tomato, sliced

Directions

1. Heat up your waffle maker.
2. Add all the chaffles Ingredients to a tiny mixing bowl and combine well.
3. Pour half of the batter into your waffle maker and cook for 4 minutes until brown. Repeat now with the rest of the batter to make another chaffle.
4. In a tiny bowl mix now the crabmeat with mayonnaise and lemon juice.
5. Top the chaffle with lettuce, tomato and the crabmeat mixture. Cover with another chaffle.
6. Serve and enjoy!

Grilled Chaffles Sandwich & Vegetables

Preparation: 5 minutes

Cooking: 12 minutes

Servings: 2 chaffles

Ingredients

For Chaffles:

- 1 large egg, beaten
- ½ cup of cheddar cheese, shredded
- ¼ tsp dried oregano

For filling:

- 1 tbsp butter
- 1 slice of American cheese
- 2 slices of grilled onions
- 2 slices of grilled zucchinis

Directions

1. Heat up your waffle maker.
2. Add all the chaffles Ingredients to a tiny mixing bowl and stir until well combined.

3. Pour half of the batter into your waffle maker and cook for 4 minutes until golden brown. Repeat now with the rest of the batter to make another chaffle.

4. Top the chaffle with a slice of American cheese, onions and zucchinis. Cover with another chaffle.

5. In a tiny saucepan, over low heat, melt the butter and cook the chaffle part by part for about 2 minutes or until the filling is Melt now.

6. Serve and enjoy!

Lemon Sauce Chicken Chaffles Sandwich

Preparation: 5 minutes

Cooking: 18 minutes

Servings: 2 chaffles

Ingredients

<u>For Chaffles:</u>

- 1 large egg, beaten
- ½ cup cheddar cheese, shredded

<u>For chicken:</u>

- ½ cup of chicken breast, shredded
- ¼ tsp garlic powder
- ¼ tsp paprika powder
- 1 tsp lemon juice
- A pinch of salt and black pepper
- 2 tbsp heavy cream
- 1 tbsp finely grated Parmesan cheese
- ½ tsp fresh thyme, minced
- ½ tsp fresh parsley, minced
- 1 tbsp unsalted butter

- ½ cup chicken broth

For filling:

- Fresh spinach leaves
- 1 tiny tomato, sliced

Directions

For chicken:

1. In a saucepan over medium heat, cook the chicken breast in the unsalted butter part by part, for approx. 10 minutes. Season with a pinch of salt, black pepper and paprika.
2. Set aside the meat.
3. In the same saucepan, add garlic powder, chicken broth, heavy cream, parmesan cheese, lemon juice and thyme. Bring to a boil and simmer until the sauce thickens. Add the chicken and mix well.

For Chaffles:

4. Heat up your waffle maker.
5. Add all the chaffles Ingredients to a tiny mixing bowl and stir until well combined.
6. Pour half of the batter into your waffle maker and cook for 4 minutes until golden brown. Repeat now with the rest of the batter to make another chaffle.

7. Top the chaffle with spinach leaves, tomato, and lemon sauce chicken. Cover with another chaffle.
8. Serve warm and enjoy!

Sliced Beef Chaffles Sandwich

Preparation: 5 minutes

Cooking: 8 minutes

Servings: 2 chaffles

Ingredients

For Chaffles:

- 1 large egg, beaten
- ½ cup mozzarella cheese, shredded

For filling:

- 1 slice of beef (seared in butter)
- 1 tbsp of keto mustard
- A pinch of black pepper
- 2 slices of grilled bell peppers
- ½ tbsp scallion, browned and chopped

Directions

For Chaffles:

1. Heat up your waffle maker.

2. Add all the chaffles Ingredients to a tiny mixing bowl and stir until well combined.
3. Pour half of the batter into your waffle maker and cook for 4 minutes until golden brown. Repeat now with the rest of the batter to make another chaffle.
4. Spread the chaffle with keto mustard, top with sliced beef, bell peppers and scallion.
5. Season with black pepper according to your taste. Cover with another chaffle.
6. Serve immediately and enjoy!

Fried Fish & Peppers Chaffles Sandwich

Preparation: 5 minutes

Cooking: 8 minutes

Servings: 2 chaffles

Ingredients

For Chaffles:

- 1 large egg, beaten
- ½ cup of mozzarella cheese, shredded
- 2 tbsp almond flour
- ¼ tsp baking powder
- 1 tbsp red bell pepper, minced
- 1 tbsp yellow bell pepper, minced
- 1 tsp fresh parsley, minced

For filling:

- Lettuce leaves
- 1 tbsp keto ketchup
- 1 fried white fish cutlet

Directions

1. Heat up your waffle maker.
2. Add all the chaffles Ingredients to a tiny mixing bowl and combine well.
3. Pour half of the batter into your waffle maker and cook for 4 minutes until brown. Repeat now with the rest of the batter to make another chaffle.
4. Spread the chaffle with ketchup and top it with lettuce and fried fish cutlet. Cover with another chaffle.
5. Serve warm and enjoy!

Cheese Peppers Chaffles Sandwich

Preparation: 5 minutes

Cooking: 8 minutes

Servings: 2 chaffles

Ingredients

For Chaffles:

- 1 large egg, beaten
- ½ cup of mozzarella cheese, shredded
- 2 tbsp almond flour
- ¼ tsp baking powder
- 1 tsp fresh parsley, minced

For filling:

- 1 tbsp keto mayonnaise
- ½ tbsp red bell pepper, grilled and thinly sliced
- ½ tbsp yellow bell pepper, grilled and thinly sliced
- Fresh spinach leaves
- 1 slice cheddar cheese

Directions

1. Heat up your waffle maker.
2. Add all the chaffles Ingredients to a tiny mixing bowl and combine well.
3. Pour half of the batter into your waffle maker and cook for 4 minutes until brown. Repeat now with the rest of the batter to make another chaffle.
4. Spread the chaffle with mayonnaise and top it with spinach leaves, cheddar cheese and peppers. Cover with another chaffle.
5. Serve warm and enjoy!

Chaffles Sandwich Ham & Guacamole

Preparation: 15 minutes

Cooking: 8 minutes

Servings: 2 chaffles

Ingredients

For the Chaffles:

- 1 cup cheddar cheese, grated
- 2 eggs, beaten
- A pinch of salt
- 1 slice ham for the filling

For Guacamole sauce:

- 1 tiny avocado pulp, mashed
- 1 tbsp cherry tomatoes, diced
- 1 tsp onions, sliced
- 2 tbsp olive oil
- 1 tbsp lemon juice
- A pinch of salt and pepper
- A pinch of Chili powder

Directions

For Guacamole sauce:

1. In a tiny bowl, add the olive oil and lemon juice to the avocado and stir.
2. Add onions, and tomatoes, mix well and season with salt, pepper, and chili to taste.

For the Chaffles:

1. Heat up your waffle maker.
2. Add all the chaffles Ingredients except ham to a tiny mixing bowl. Stir until well combined.
3. Pour half of the batter into your waffle maker and cook for 4 minutes. Repeat now with the rest of the batter to make another chaffle.
4. Spread the guacamole on a chaffle and cover with ham, then put another chaffle on top.
5. Serve and enjoy!

Swiss Cheese and Salami Chaffles Sandwich

Preparation: 5 minutes

Cooking: 8 minutes

Servings: 2 chaffles

Ingredients

For Chaffles:

- 1 large egg, beaten
- ½ cup of Swiss cheese, shredded

For filling:

- 1-2 slices of Salami
- 1 tbsp keto Ranch dressing
- Lettuce leaves

Directions

1. Heat up your waffle maker.
2. Add all the chaffles Ingredients to a tiny mixing bowl and combine well.

3. Pour half of the batter into your waffle maker and cook for 4 minutes until golden brown. Repeat now with the rest of the batter to make another chaffle.
4. Let cool for 3 minutes to let chaffles get crispy.
5. Spread the chaffle with Ranch dressing. Top the chaffle with lettuce and a slice of Salami. Cover with another chaffle.
6. Serve and enjoy!

Strawberry Cream Sandwich Chaffles

Preparation: 6 minutes

Cooking: 6 Minutes

Servings: 2

Ingredients

Chaffles:

- 1 large organic egg, beaten
- ½ cup mozzarella cheese, shredded finely

Filling:

- 4 teaspns heavy cream
- 2 tbsps powdered erythritol
- 1 teaspn fresh lemon juice
- Pinch of fresh lemon zest, grated
- 2 fresh strawberries, hulled and sliced

Directions

1. Preheat now a waffle iron and then grease it.
2. For chaffles, add the egg and mozzarella cheese and stir to combine in a tiny bowl.

3. Place half of the mixture into Preheat waffle iron and cook for about 2–minutes.
4. Repeat now with the remaining mixture.
5. Meanwhile, for filling: in a bowl, place all the Ingredients except the strawberry slices and with a hand mixer, beat until well combined.
6. Serve each chaffle with cream mixture and strawberry slices.

Nutrition:

Calories: 140, Fat: 1.1g, Carbs: 27.9g, Protein: 4.7g, Fiber: 10.9g

Spicy Flavored Chaffle

Preparation: 5 min

Cooking: 4 min

Servings: 2

Ingredients

- 1 cup Cheddar cheese (shredded)
- 1 large Egg
- 1 oz Cream cheese
- 2 tbsp Bacon bits
- 2 Jalapenos, sliced
- 1/4 tsp Baking powder (optional)

Directions

1. Preheat now the waffle maker until hot
2. Whisk egg in a bowl, add cheese, then mix well
3. Stir in the remaining Ingredients (except toppings, if any).
4. Scoop 1/2 of the batter onto your waffle maker, spread across evenly
5. Cook 3-4 min, until done as desired (or crispy).

6. Gently Remove now from waffle maker and let it cool
7. Repeat now with remaining batter.
8. Top with Melt cheese, jalapeno slices, and bacon bits

Nutrition:

231 Calories, 2g Net Carbs, 18g Fat, 13g Protein

Keto Chaffle With Cream

Preparation: 5 min

Cooking: 4 min

Servings: 2

Ingredients

- 1 large egg
- 1/2 cup shredded mozzarella
- 1 tbsp of almond flour
- 1 tsp vanilla
- 1 shake of cinnamon
- 1/2 tsp baking powder
- 1/2 tbsp whipped cream

Directions

1. Preheat now the waffle maker until hot
2. Whisk egg in a bowl, add cheese, then mix well
3. Stir in the remaining Ingredients (except toppings, if any).
4. Scoop ½ of the batter on your waffle maker, spread across evenly
5. Cook until a bit browned and crispy, about 4 minutes.

6. Cook 3-4 min, until done as desired (or crispy).
7. Gently Remove now from waffle maker and let it cool
8. Repeat now with remaining batter.
9. Top with whipped cream and cinnamon

Nutrition:

271 Calories, 2g Net Carbs, 27g Fat, 13g Protein

Sweet & Spicy Chaffle

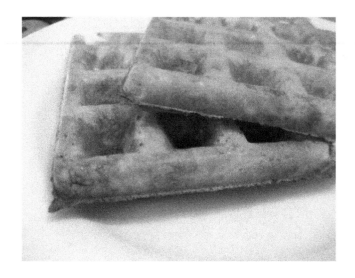

Preparation: 5 min

Cooking: 4 min

Servings: 2

Ingredients

- 1 large egg
- 1/2 cup mozzarella cheese
- 2 tbsp Stevia, liquid
- 1/2 tsp salt
- 1/2 tsp smoked paprika

- Pinch of cayenne pepper

Directions

1. Preheat now the waffle maker until hot
2. Whisk egg in a bowl, add cheese, then mix well
3. Stir in the remaining Ingredients (except toppings, if any).
4. Scoop 1/2 of the batter onto your waffle maker, spread across evenly
5. Cook 3-4 min, until done as desired (or crispy).
6. Gently Remove now from waffle maker and let it cool
7. Repeat now with remaining batter.
8. Top with whipped cream and cinnamon

Nutrition:

252 Calories, 3g Net Carbs, 21g Fat, 12g Protein

Savory Herb Chaffle

Preparation: 5 min

Cooking: 4 min

Servings: 2

Ingredients

- 1 large egg
- 1/4 cup shredded mozzarella
- 1/4 cup shredded parmesan
- 1/2 tbsp butter, Melt
- 1 tsp herb blend seasoning
- 1/2 tsp salt

Directions

1. Preheat now the waffle maker until hot
2. Whisk egg in a bowl, add cheese, then mix well
3. Stir in the remaining Ingredients (except toppings, if any).
4. Scoop 1/2 of the batter onto your waffle maker, spread across evenly

5. Cook until a bit browned and crispy, about 4 minutes.

6. Cook 3-4 min, until done as desired (or crispy).

7. Gently Remove now from waffle maker and let it cool

8. Repeat now with remaining batter.

9. Serve and Enjoy!

Nutrition:

294 Calories, 2g Net Carbs, 24g Fat, 12g Protein

Hot Brown Sandwich Chaffle

Preparation: 15 minutes

Cooking: 5 minutes

Servings: 2

Ingredients

For the Chaffles:

- 1 egg, beaten
- 1/4 cup cheddar cheese, shredded and divided

For the Sandwich:

- 2 slices fresh tomato
- 1/2 lb roasted turkey breast
- 1/2 tsp parmesan cheese, grated
- 2 bacon, cooked

For the sauce:

- 2 oz cream cheese, cubed
- 1/3 cup of heavy cream
- 1/4 cup swiss cheese, shredded
- 1/4 tsp ground nutmeg
- White pepper

Directions

1. Preheat now your waffle maker.
2. Start by making the chaffle, once heated up, sprinkle 1 tbsp cheddar cheese onto the iron.
3. After 30 seconds, top the cheese with beaten egg.
4. Once the egg starts to cook, top the mixture with another cheese layer.
5. Close your waffle maker lid and allow to cook for 3-5 minutes until the chaffle is crispy and golden brown.
6. Take out the cooked chaffle and repeat the steps until you've used up all the batter.
7. Make the sauce by combining heavy cream and cream cheese in a tiny saucepan.
8. Place saucepan over medium heat and whisk until the cheese completely dissolves.
9. Add in Swiss cheese and parmesan, then continue whisking to Melt now the cheese.
10. Add in the white pepper and nutmeg.
11. Continue whisking until you achieve a smooth consistency.
12. Remove now the sauce pan from heat.
13. Prepare the sandwich by setting the oven for broiling.
14. Cover a cookie sheet with aluminum foil.

15. Lightly grease the foil with butter, and place two chaffles on it.
16. Top the chaffles with 4 oz of turkey and a slice of tomato each. Add some sauce and grated parmesan on top.
17. Broil the chaffle sandwiches for 2-3 minutes until you see the sauce bubble and brown spots appear on top.
18. Remove now from the oven. Put them on a heatproof plate.
19. Arrange bacon slices in a crisscross manner on top of the sandwich before serving.

Nutrition:

Calories: 572, Carbohydrates: 3g, Fat: 41g, Protein: 41g

CPSIA information can be obtained
at www.ICGtesting.com
Printed in the USA
BVHW091048090621
609091BV00008B/722